1.50

THE TRY SOFTER GUIDED JOURNEY

THE
TRY SOFTER
GUIDED JOURNEY

A Soulful Companion to Healing

AUNDI KOLBER MA LPC

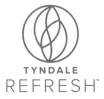

TYNDALE
REFRESH™
Think Well. Live Well. Be Well.

Visit Tyndale online at tyndale.com.

Tyndale and Tyndale's quill logo are registered trademarks of Tyndale House Ministries. *Tyndale Refresh* and the Tyndale Refresh logo are trademarks of Tyndale House Ministries. Tyndale Refresh is a nonfiction imprint of Tyndale House Publishers, Carol Stream, Illinois.

The Try Softer Guided Journey: A Soulful Companion to Healing

Copyright © 2021 by Andrea M. Kolber. All rights reserved.

Cover illustration by Eva M. Winters. Copyright © Tyndale House Ministries. All rights reserved.

Cover photograph of texture copyright © korkeng/Adobe Stock. All rights reserved.

Author photo taken by Ben Haley, copyright © 2019. All rights reserved.

Designed by Eva M. Winters

Published in association with Don Gates of the literary agency The Gates Group; www.the-gates-group.com.

Scripture quotation marked KJV is taken from the *Holy Bible*, King James Version.

Scripture quotations marked NIV are taken from the Holy Bible, *New International Version*,® *NIV*.® Copyright © 1973, 1978, 1984, 2011 by Biblica, Inc.® Used by permission. All rights reserved worldwide.

Scripture quotations marked MSG are taken from *The Message*, copyright © 1993, 2002, 2018 by Eugene H. Peterson. Used by permission of NavPress. All rights reserved. Represented by Tyndale House Publishers.

For information about special discounts for bulk purchases, please contact Tyndale House Publishers at csresponse@tyndale.com, or call 1-855-277-9400.

ISBN 978-1-4964-5467-6

Printed in the United States of America

27	26	25	24	23	22	21
7	6	5	4	3	2	1

CONTENTS

INTRODUCTION

THE OTHER MORNING I AWOKE BEFORE THE SUN. An anxious thought was twirling in my mind and wouldn't quit reverberating. It wasn't about anything I could actually change, mind you. Just one of those pesky in-between-sleep-and-consciousness ideas. Though it was a Saturday and I had no need to wake for some time, I almost decided to get out of bed just to make it stop. Then as I sat up in a morning haze, a calm inner voice said, *It's okay, Aundi. You don't need to figure it out right now. You can rest.*

Wordlessly, I laid my head back on the pillow and felt my body exhale as sleep found me once again.

Truth be told, I'm not sure whether the voice I heard was from the Spirit or my own compassionate inner self. These days, they work together quite frequently. Regardless, it was exactly what I needed in those early morning hours. Later that day I shared the experience with my husband, Brendan, and tears unexpectedly filled my eyes. For me, seeing the continuation of all the ways we can heal and move toward wholeness felt like a tiny Ebenezer of God's faithfulness. I don't think there will ever be a time when I won't feel deep gratitude for learning to show up differently in the world.

Learning to try softer—that is, to cultivate compassionate attention for our whole selves—has been a crucial element of that healing. Even as I write today, our country is neck-deep in a global pandemic, issues of racial injustice, and political unrest—and for the first time ever, my husband and I are considering homeschooling. We are grateful and privileged to have the opportunity to consider how we educate our kiddos. Yet it's all still a bit overwhelming. In the midst of so much individual and collective turmoil, I'm finding that I need the message of "try softer" more than ever. I need to remember it's okay to honor and attend to the information my body gives me. I need to recall that my value is not, and has never been, based on what I produce. It's essential I remember that embodying a gentle posture with myself allows me to more deeply and attentively love others in my life too.

The reality is, I won't ever graduate from trying softer. This is the work of my life—of being alive. And this, too, is grace. It is a gift to know we are constantly invited into a compassionate posture, not so we can stay stuck, but so we can live into who God created us to be. And while it may seem like a paradox, I believe now is exactly the time when we need to cultivate tenderness and compassion for the pain that exists in the world—not only for others but also for ourselves.

I want this for you, too, dear one. If you're reading these words, you're likely on the same path as I am: a nonlinear journey of hard-earned steps toward wholeness, compassion, and inner healing. Whether you've read *Try Softer* and feel ready to dig deeper into its principles or you've been doing this work for a while and are looking for more guided support, I welcome you. I hope you see these pages as a gentle and accessible invitation to further learning. I pray this work feels like an exhale to your soul, and that you, too, can learn to be with yourself differently. And most of all, I hope that when tender wounds from your life surface, you'll steward grace toward them in the same way our good God already does.

A GENTLE GUIDE

If you'll allow me to be blunt, I'm not typically a big fan of workbooks. I know, I know . . . here I am writing one. But here's why I've tended to stay away from them in the past: They don't always lend themselves to the flexibility that's needed to attune to each of our stories, bodies, and spirits. The questions or exercises presented can sometimes feel like rigid tasks we have to complete even if they feel overwhelming, like measures or standards we *have* to meet by the end of the book in order to truly heal. And as you may know from reading *Try Softer*, white-knuckling like this—forcing ourselves to engage when our bodies and spirits don't feel safe to do so—often only ends in staying stuck, or at worst, experiencing further trauma and pain.

With this in mind, you will notice that I do all that I can to give you as much choice as possible as you engage with this material. This is not by accident. As we talk about in *Try Softer*, choice is crucial to learning to pay compassionate attention to oneself; as you move through this content, I want you to feel free to make it work for you.

In each session, you'll find several invitations to help you more deeply process the content—invitations that are designed to engage and explore your inner world, your creativity, and your hopes for the future. As much as you're able, listen to the information and wisdom that your body is communicating, and honor that. Give yourself permission to go slow; if you feel overwhelmed, you can skip questions—even entire sections!—and come back to them if or when you can.

Trying softer can be empowering, freeing, and life-giving. And yet some elements of the journey can be difficult, deep, and heavy. My prayer is that the words and practices ahead will empower you for the fullness of the *sacred* work before you. May this guided journey be a gentle support, a companion helping you come home to yourself as you decide the route and set the pace for your journey.

Here's a more detailed look at what you can expect along the way.

Holding Space for Our Stories

One of the most beautiful concepts I've come to learn, both professionally and personally, is that stories change and move us. Not only that; we also carry our own stories of lived experiences in our bodies. At the beginning of each session, to help us more deeply combine and integrate concepts from *Try Softer*, you'll find a short personal reflection to help you continue processing concepts learned in the corresponding *Try Softer* chapters. You can also find free, short video introductions for each of these sessions on my website—aundikolber.com/videos.

Body-Centered Exercise

The work we do in *Try Softer*—it's not for the faint of heart. It can be hard and painful, deep soul work that requires compassion and gentleness. We learned in *Try Softer* how to check in with ourselves and our bodies, and while I invite you to do this throughout the guide, each session will also have space to explicitly focus on our bodies. These practices are an extension of what you'll have learned in the corresponding chapters of *Try Softer* and are meant to help you more deeply anchor the content we're working through in your whole self. With that said, safety is key: You'll notice that I often provide cues to make sure we're accessing body work in a way and pace that feels doable to you. Please know that regardless of the extent to which you engage in the practices I provide, by just honoring the pace of your body, you are already beginning to try softer.

Invitation to Reflect and Discuss

While much of the work we do with trying softer is individual, we also know that God wired our bodies for interpersonal connection and coregulation. If you want to do this work in an authentic and supportive group environment, you can adapt and facilitate accordingly. These questions are meant to spark introspection and reflection—as well as conversation and sharing to the extent that you feel comfortable. Because this is such vulnerable and personal work, I've included a short guide, "Guidance for Group Leaders," in the back of this book to highlight core components of trauma-informed communication. Especially in groups, creating and maintaining safety is of utmost importance. Be intentional about cultivating a space of trust—and give each other permission to participate and interact with the material *as you personally choose to.* You are the best judge of how much of your story and your experience feels helpful to disclose. My hope is that hearing that you are not alone on this journey of trying softer will be a balm of encouragement to your soul.

Invitation to Journal

Much of the deep work of compassionate attention happens squarely within your mind, body, and psyche—and this journaling section is one way to continue to attune to your own story. Many of the prompts I've written for you here are similar to questions and activities I would delve into if we were sitting in my therapy office. My hope is that as you engage with these questions, they will provide a springboard toward gently holding and honoring the complexities of your personhood.

Invitation to Create

Have you ever noticed that some experiences are hard to describe with words? Or have you ever felt like words weren't enough? This can happen to all of us from time to time, but it can be especially true when parts of our stories have been distressing or traumatic. This is why I want to invite you to use art to gently tap into your right brain, which researchers note is connected to imagery, symbolism, emotion, and sensation.[1] Even when parts of our stories aren't distressing, finding ways to access the right brain can be helpful for continuing to move toward integration and wholeness—for it is from a place of deeper integration that we can continue to pay compassionate attention to the wounds that are still aching.

In the "Invitation to Create" section, you'll find a few ideas for prompts. As always, feel free to adapt these so they best empower you as you honor your story. And as a sidenote, many of us wouldn't consider ourselves artists, and that's okay! As with all our work, the process of creating is as important as what we've created, no matter how it turns out.

Reader, if I could look into your eyes at this exact moment, this is what I'd say: "I am so proud of you. I am proud that you are willing to engage in this sacred work." Having counseled many folks and walked on this path for many years myself, I know it's not easy to lean in where it aches. My greatest and audacious hope for you, dear one, is that the work ahead will help you sink deeper into the truthiest truth I know: You are beloved. And because that's true, you can come to these pages knowing that no matter what your story holds, you are already loved by the God of the universe. May this give you profound courage, and may it ground you in goodness as you grow.

YOU

ARE

BELOVED

THE GOAL OF TRYING SOFTER

ISN'T TO BRING ABOUT A QUICK FIX, BUT TO

EMPOWER US WITH THE FREEDOM TO LIVE IN

THE HERE & NOW WHILE STILL HONORING

& TENDING TO THE WOUNDS OF OUR STORIES

THAT HAVE KEPT US DISCONNECTED FROM

OUR EXPERIENCES.

TRY SOFTER, PAGE 20

THE STORIES WE HOLD
IN OUR BODIES

A Deeper Dive into Chapters 1 and 2 of *Try Softer*

SEVERAL YEARS AGO when I worked with a young woman named Lindsey,[1] she would come into our sessions explaining how excited she was to be in therapy. Some of her friends had given her feedback that at times she seemed disconnected from her emotions, and she wanted to fix that. She wasn't an emotional person, she declared, but she often got heartburn or stomachaches when life was intense. During our initial intake, Lindsey often summarized her family when she was growing up as "pretty perfect" and "super support-ive." However, as we processed together in the sessions that followed, Lindsey's emotions curiously remained flat as she shared how "great" her parents were.

Once, as we neared the holidays, I asked Lindsey about how her family celebrated together.

"Hmm," she mused thoughtfully. "Well, I was such a deep feeler as a kid. My mom says I cried all the time. I think it drove my parents nuts. In fact, my dog died when I was eight, and I nearly ruined Christmas because of it."

"Can you tell me more, Lindsey? What do you mean when you say you 'nearly ruined Christmas'?" I asked.

"Well, when I found out how Max had died, I started crying, and I, well, I guess I couldn't stop. We had to get to church, so my dad started yelling at me," Lindsey recalled. "Gosh, I really messed that night up. I can't believe I overreacted so much. My dad really didn't like it when I cried, and I'm pretty sure he didn't like Max that much." She shrugged matter-of-factly. "So yeah, I mean, pretty typical stuff."

"Lindsey," I said to her, as her face remained stoic, "the story you just told me about your family feels incredibly sad—and I'm honored that you'd share it with me—but I'm noticing you don't seem to have any emotion about it. While you are the only one who can identify what you're feeling, I'm curious to see if there may be something else going on in your body as you share it."

"Hmmm. I mean, yeah, I see what you mean. It is a sad story, but I just feel disconnected from it. I guess I feel like I should just be over it by now," Lindsey explained.

"Okay—would you be willing to try something with me for a second?" I asked her.

"Sure," she said, nodding.

"Could you take a moment and scan your body, and as you do, can you tell me if you're noticing any sensations or emotions?" I asked.

As Lindsey did, she shared with me that she felt almost nothing in her body at all. Which, as discussed on pages 32–33 in *Try Softer*, is in itself important and helpful information about Lindsey's nervous system. As she talked, I tracked and closely attuned to Lindsey's body language; as a therapist, this is one of the most important ways I can listen. I said something that felt quite bold at the time, but I had a hunch it was accurate.

"Lindsey, feel free to reject this if it doesn't resonate—but are you sensing any heat or tension in your upper chest?" I asked.

The room was quiet for twenty to thirty seconds before she answered, "Yes, yes, I am. Wait—what? That's strange . . ."

I asked Lindsey if she could assign an emotion to the sensation she was feeling, and finally she was able to say that a mixture of sadness and shame was coming up for her.

It was a turning point. As our work continued, Lindsey gained the tolerance and skill to be with her body differently and to recognize that her experiences from childhood were significant not just twenty years ago, but even now in the ways her body continued to express her pain. Eventually Lindsey was able to grieve and process the fact that her parents often shamed her for her emotions and the way it shaped her inability to feel emotions in her present-day life.

Our bodies *do* communicate with us; even if we *feel* disconnected, our bodies are holding and witnessing the experiences of our lives—and if we can learn to listen, if we can learn to speak the language of our bodies, we can unlock a whole new understanding of how we move through the world. I talk a lot about my own story in *Try Softer*, how I white-knuckled and ignored what my body was telling me in order to survive. It's not to say all those experiences from my childhood were bad, but I was often on my own emotionally. White-knuckling became my default reaction—my body did everything it could to get me through a childhood peppered with interpersonal trauma.

My own healing work has centered on finding ways to be grateful for my body, grateful that I was able to figure out how to survive. Even now, I recall with fondness the younger me who truly was doing her best without the kind of support she needed. You see, I didn't have a choice but to be strong; this is why at that time I had to push myself so hard. But white-knuckling your way through life is akin to having a carrot on a string placed in front of you, while never being able to touch it. You never arrive; it's never enough.

I realize that it's incredibly simple to write these words, and a whole different thing to live them. It's easy for me to tell you that we don't have to white-knuckle our way through our lives. It's an entirely different—and more difficult—posture to extend that compassion to myself in moments when I am living as though I were defined by my old narratives.

Sometimes learning the language of our bodies and confronting our stories in this new way can feel scary. It can seem easier to continue white-knuckling our way through life, pushing and pushing; even though we're disconnected, at least we're surviving, right? If we embrace our stories and allow ourselves to feel our feelings, admitting that we're overwhelmed, does that make us weak?

Dear heart, let me assure you—it does not. God is tremendously kind to us and doesn't shame us for our inability to be less than human. Paradoxically, I've learned that our capacity to be with ourselves and our stories is part of what allows us to pay compassionate attention to our experiences. This is why honoring the process matters so deeply; it paves the way for the truest healing.

BODY-CENTERED EXERCISE

When we notice that we're overwhelmed or disconnected from our bodies as we engage with our stories, one practice we can employ is reaching for things that bring us comfort and ground us in the present moment.

For this exercise, you'll create your own sensory toolbox to have on hand—a collection of some of your favorite things. As you fill your sensory toolbox,[2] think about what feels nurturing to you, what you can focus on to bring you back to the moment after doing the hard work of embracing your story. In my own life, I've learned there are a few tried-and-true treasures that ground me when I'm feeling overwhelmed. If it helps, imagine me doing this work with you as I gather my own nurturing items: decaf chai tea, eucalyptus essential oil, several ridged seashells from the Oregon coast, a beige candle, Sandra McCracken's music playing in the background, and finally—a picture of the Pacific Ocean. And in case you need a reminder, you're worth this kind of care, dear one.

Here are some ideas for your Try Softer sensory toolbox:

Taste: gum, mints, tea, etc.

Sight: a picture or written words reflecting something that is soothing or nurturing, such as a photo, painting, poetry, Bible verse, or quote. (I love the ocean, so I put a picture of that in my toolbox!)

Hearing: instrumental music, hymns, a sound machine, a voice recording or podcast, etc.

Smell: essential oils, a tea bag, herbs, etc.

Touch: flannel, silk, a rock, sand, sculpting clay, etc.

Throughout our journey together, you can feel free to use your sensory toolbox at any point. Please remember you don't have to wait until you're overwhelmed to utilize this resource—it can be a form of ongoing self-care!

INVITATION TO REFLECT AND DISCUSS

1. Where do you see that you may be white-knuckling in your life right now? How do you know?

2. Do you have a sense of what has kept you from engaging with your story until now? If you can, briefly summarize what those reasons might be. Feel free to use one-word descriptions such as *trust* or *support* if this topic feels too overwhelming to dive into.

3. What does it mean to embrace your story? What does safely embracing your story look like in your life?

4. On pages 13–14 of *Try Softer*, I tell the story of Erica, who journeys to find the spaces of her story where she learned to avoid or minimize pain. How does this kind of avoidance show up in your life? Take note of the specific situations where you find yourself frequently minimizing your own experience.

5. What parts of your story do you struggle to believe really matter? What's one step you can take to begin the journey of embracing your story?

6. On page 15 of *Try Softer*, I say, "The stories we weave and the meaning we make from them create templates for how we understand God, life, others, and ourselves." In what ways does your story color your experience of God?

7. Where in your story do you feel proud of yourself for what you've made it through or how you've adapted to change?

8. How do you feel when you're hyperaroused, or in "fight/flight/fawn[3] mode"? What about when you're hypoaroused, or in "freeze mode"?

9. My definition of trauma is broad and wide-reaching. On page 34 of *Try Softer*, I define trauma as "anything that overwhelms a person's nervous system and ability to cope." While big T trauma tends to be more obvious (and certainly requires care), sometimes little t trauma is overlooked and minimized. Do you feel like you've had instances of little t trauma in your story? If so, spend time reflecting on those instances to the extent that feels helpful to you. How does your body respond to the reframing of your story through the lens of trauma? See the graphic on the following page for helpful prompts.

Big T Trauma

Witnessing or experiencing any of the following events can result in post-traumatic stress disorder:*

- a life-threatening situation
- sexual violence
- serious injury
- natural disaster

I may experience or feel:

- triggered by anything that reminds me of the event;
- emotional or visual flashbacks that bring up the same emotions or sensations as during the event;
- a desire to avoid thoughts or feelings related to the event;
- nervous system dysregulation (anxiety/depression/anger/fear related to the event); or
- a change in core belief about myself related to the event (e.g., I'm bad; It's my fault).

Little t Trauma

Little t trauma includes any experience that overwhelms your ability to cope and continues to feel disturbing, situations such as

- being the target of bullying;
- having absent/estranged parents;
- being the target of verbal/emotional abuse;
- going through a bad breakup;
- experiencing racism or discrimination;
- experiencing grief or loss;
- experiencing intense transitions;
- growing up in poverty; or
- undergoing medical procedures.

*Please keep in mind that this is not meant as the full diagnostic criteria for PTSD. If you suspect you may have PTSD, please see a mental health professional for a full evaluation.

10. What does it feel like (physically or emotionally) to be disconnected from your body?

11. Reflect on a time when you felt like you weren't just surviving—you were truly *thriving*. What were the circumstances? What do you notice in your body as you remember that time?

INVITATION TO JOURNAL

As you are comfortable, write out the scene of a time when you white-knuckled your way through something. I encourage you to get as descriptive as possible to really put yourself in the moment. This way, you can begin to become more aware of how you uniquely respond to stressors and overwhelm. (If at any time this exercise feels overwhelming, you may always stop and/or utilize your sensory toolbox to bring you back to the present in a nurturing way.) As you write, take a moment to notice your body. What do you observe? Does it feel tight, warm, tingly, etc.? For now, just notice.

If you feel able, take a moment and pause to consider the reality that your body has been working hard to keep you safe and protected your entire life (even when you haven't felt that way!). God designed our bodies to need and want safety, and this is important and necessary. For many of us, this essential safety was lacking in childhood or in other important relationships later on. When those basic emotional or physical needs are not met, we are designed to adapt in the best way we know how—which may result in experiences like Lindsey's from the beginning reflection. This is a completely normal reaction in the context. When you've finished, I invite you to take a moment and place your hand on your heart, stomach, or head and simply acknowledge—either out loud or to yourself—the work they have done. As you do this, simply notice what it's like to pause.

INVITATION TO CREATE

Take a moment to pull out the timeline you were asked to create on page 21 of *Try Softer*. Pick an event on the timeline, and give yourself permission to draw a picture about the event as you're able. As you do, consider what colors you are drawn to and whether there are shapes or images that feel appropriate for what you're expressing. Do you want to take up a lot of space or a little on the page?

Another option to consider for this exercise is to draw the entire arc of your story artistically, almost like a bird's-eye view of your entire experience. As with the first option, consider what colors you are drawn to. Are they dark or light? How much of the page do you want to take up? Would it include people, or would it focus more on a place?

Finally, as you create, I want to invite you to be mindful of your body. Are you tense or relaxed? Notice if you feel grounded or disconnected. As always, you can engage to the extent that feels helpful for you.

I HOPE YOU FIND

SOMEONE WHO SPEAKS

YOUR LANGUAGE SO YOU DON'T

HAVE TO SPEND A LIFETIME

TRANSLATING YOUR SPIRIT.

DR. THEMA BRYANT-DAVIS

CONNECTION IS THE CURRENCY OF REGULATION

A Deeper Dive into Chapters 3 and 4 of *Try Softer*

IT HAD BEEN A DAY.

You know what I mean, right? Nothing had gone well. Someone I trusted had hurt me. Everything seemed broken. I had made several mistakes, snapped at my children more than I care to admit, and felt like my heart was going to beat out of my chest—while simultaneously feeling frozen in place and like I couldn't catch my breath. In a situation like this, a younger me might have taken all this information my body was giving me and then shamed myself for being so weak. Next, I might have told myself to stuff it down (until I perhaps exploded with anger or experienced another way my body was trying to get my attention).

It's fair to say I was feeling many big emotions that day, and I was definitely beginning to move outside my window of tolerance (WOT). I discuss this concept at length in chapter 4 of *Try Softer*. Essentially, our WOT speaks to the range of arousal our nervous system can experience before moving into either fight/flight/fawn or freeze.[1] Once we are completely outside our WOT, we no longer have access to our prefrontal cortex, which is the part of the brain that helps us stay fully connected to our body, mind, and spirit. This is also the element of our brain that allows us to observe our experience so we can pay compassionate attention.

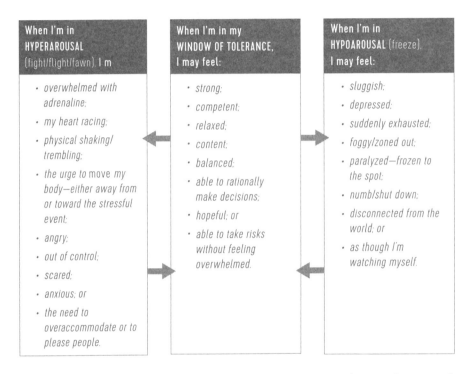

When I'm in HYPERAROUSAL (fight/flight/fawn), I m	When I'm in my WINDOW OF TOLERANCE, I may feel:	When I'm in HYPOAROUSAL (freeze), I may feel:
• overwhelmed with adrenaline;	• strong;	• sluggish;
• my heart racing;	• competent;	• depressed;
• physical shaking/ trembling;	• relaxed;	• suddenly exhausted;
• the urge to move my body—either away from or toward the stressful event;	• content;	• foggy/zoned out;
	• balanced;	• paralyzed—frozen to the spot;
• angry;	• able to rationally make decisions;	• numb/shut down;
• out of control;	• hopeful; or	• disconnected from the world; or
• scared;	• able to take risks without feeling overwhelmed.	• as though I'm watching myself.
• anxious; or		
• the need to overaccommodate or to please people.		

Reader, I told you that story partly because it happened just a few months ago. Even after all the work I've done, there are still times that are just plain hard. There are times when my body still naturally wants to white-knuckle.

Yet here's what made the difference on that particular day: I knew it was okay to have a hard time and ask for help. As Brené Brown says, "What we don't need in the midst of struggle is shame for being human." Can I get an amen? After years of practicing, I was able to remember just how much attachment matters. I remembered that often leaning into the strength and resources of at least one other trusted nervous system—a friend, spouse, or family member—can make all the difference in terms of becoming more stabilized and getting myself back to a place where I feel like my whole self.

When my husband, Brendan, got home, I said, "I don't think I'm okay. I need a hug, and then I need to go on a walk." Then I called my sister and another dear friend. I let my body move, I remembered I am beloved, and I practiced compassionate attention while I remembered I am not alone.

That night as we sat to process for a moment, both Brendan and I were exhausted. He held my hand. I cried. He lent me his strength and groundedness in that moment. I exhaled and felt tender toward the intensity of my day. We actually didn't say much; I knew it was okay to just be.

This is the power of attachment.

With attachment, we come to know we are held in the mind of another, and we hold them in our own minds.[2] And this holding allows us to be tender toward ourselves. Connection with God and others is the currency that allows each of us to experience coregulation; this is the pathway toward self-regulation and staying rooted in our own personal WOT.

This work teaches us to steward toward ourselves the love and honor we experience from others as a resource to connect with our own nervous systems. We are not simply nervous systems who exist in isolation. Instead, we are a part of a whole; our entire selves, including our nervous systems, are meant to interconnect with and influence others. We are both uniquely individual and tied together. Perhaps this is part of the reason why Jesus places such emphasis on His command to love our neighbors as ourselves. I can't help but observe He knows that how we treat ourselves and each other does indeed matter.

If you've read *Try Softer*, you know much of my own personal trauma is connected to relational and attachment trauma—which is why it's a big deal for me to know I can ask for help.

How about you, dear one? As you read through the various attachment styles in *Try Softer*, what do they bring up for you? Do you feel permission to "parent" the parts of your story that are wounded?

If this is still a work in progress for you or you are just beginning, I am so glad you are here. If you are already doing this work of tending to your pain with compassion—well done for continuing the work.

BODY-CENTERED EXERCISE

Our attachment styles are like templates that live in our bodies and are formed by a network of experiences.[3] These templates are not static but are usually rooted in our earliest experiences of care.[4] Over the course of many experiences, we come to predict how those we love will respond to us when we are in pain, alone, or in need of support.[5] With that said, part of learning to try softer in this area is becoming more acquainted with how our bodies respond to our specific attachment styles.

For this exercise, you'll be using some of what you've already practiced in *Try Softer* on pages 67–69. As you consider what your primary attachment style may be (autonomous, preoccupied, dismissive, fearful-avoidant), take a moment to scan your body and observe what you notice.

If you notice any sensations, I invite you to place your hand on that part of your body. If the attachment style itself doesn't bring up any sensations or emotions, think of a time when you were sick or needed help; then see how your body responds to that memory. For a moment, simply notice your body's response. Take a moment to see whether you can name its size, shape, and/or color. Now, if this sensation had a voice, what might it say?

For example, when I'm overwhelmed and begin to realize my need to connect with my support system, I sometimes notice a tight sensation in my throat. While the sensation and where I feel it in my body can vary, I've come to understand that it means an old wound is surfacing that originates from my history of having an anxious-ambivalent attachment style. Though I've experienced

ATTACHMENT STYLES

AUTONOMOUS

(Secure Attachment)

- *Tend to be interdependent and able to connect with others and themselves*
- *Can acknowledge their own faults while also hearing their partners' concerns*
- *Are able to stay emotionally regulated in everyday situations involving relationships*
- *Are able to more accurately assess whether a person is safe or reliable based on their previous experiences*

PREOCCUPIED

(Anxious-Ambivalent Attachment)

- *Tend to desire validation and closeness*
- *Are most afraid of abandonment*
- *Are hypercritical of self but more apt to see others as "good"*
- *Tend to be emotionally dysregulated*
- *Are typically triggered by conflict and react by wanting more closeness*
- *Experience the most engagement from their sympathetic nervous systems (fight/flight/fawn) when triggered[6]*

DISMISSIVE

(Avoidant Attachment)

- *Tend to be self-reliant*
- *Are most afraid of feeling "engulfed" by other people*
- *Tend to be critical of others but less critical of themselves*
- *Are emotionally disconnected*
- *Are typically triggered by conflict; react by isolating to try to emotionally self-regulate*
- *Experience the most engagement from their sympathetic nervous systems (fight/flight/fawn) when triggered[7]*

FEARFUL-AVOIDANT

(Disorganized Attachment)

- *Desire to connect to other people but also fear being used and hurt*
- *Are most afraid that those closest to them will cause them harm*
- *Tend to see themselves as defective and others as scary*
- *May feel they are inviting others in while also pushing them out*
- *Tend to be emotionally dysregulated, which may result in dissociation and/or sympathetic nervous system activation*
- *In relationships, may experience feelings reminiscent of the terror experienced in childhood*

significant healing, it's normal for my earliest attachment style to need tending even as I now primarily identify with having earned secure attachment.

At times when I notice this tightness in my throat, the sense I often have is that it may not be okay to ask for help because perhaps my request won't be met with follow-through or care. As I notice the sensation, I place my hand gently on my throat and recall that though my husband and others who care about me aren't perfect, they love me and want to support me. As I do this, I notice that the sensation begins to lessen. This is one example of how we can connect the work of attachment with the wisdom of our bodies.

Depending on the information you receive from this exercise, you may want to journal about it below. You could also ask the sensation/image/voice what it might need from you to feel supported.

Please be aware that for some this may be an activating exercise for the nervous system; because our attachment styles are often rooted in our relationships with our primary caregivers, we can often have visceral reactions when we engage in this work. As always, you are free to do this to the extent that feels doable for you.

INVITATION TO REFLECT AND DISCUSS

1. In your mind, what does a relationship filled with attunement and repair look like? What phrases or actions make you feel uniquely known and seen?

2. Take a moment to consider how different attachment styles affect our relationships, even with yourself and your inner child.[6] In the circles on the next page, I invite you to list words that might describe your relationship with self, God, and others. Don't worry whether they fit in clinical language or not. Simply give yourself permission to honestly assess how you experience attachment in each of these categories. For example, some may experience God, but not others, as trustworthy (or vice versa). As you're able, see where these relationships seem to overlap, or not, and note your observations.

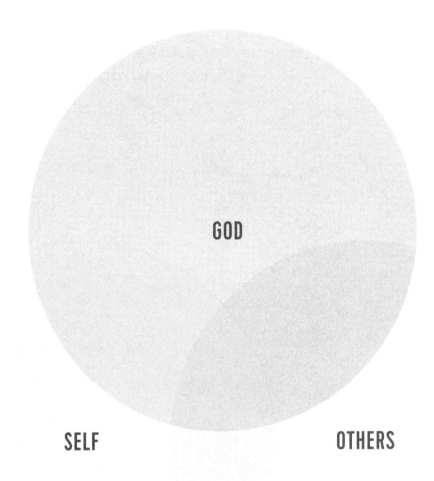

GOD

SELF   OTHERS

3. Where do you see the attachment style you formed with your caregivers show up in your relationships today? How does coming to a better understanding of your early attachment help you see these relationships in a new light?

4. The idea of internalized safety is key to forming healthy, secure attachments. What does safety feel like to you?

5. Where do you see your primary attachment style show up in your relationship with God?

6. One of the goals of attachment work is to cultivate a strong "inner voice" that can serve as the parent we needed as children. What are some affirming statements you needed to hear as a child? What are some ways you can be gentle and affirming to your inner child today? I've included a sidebar with additional ideas for reparenting statements.

REPARENTING STATEMENTS

Below is a list of reparenting statements to utilize if they are helpful to you. When considering your inner child, something to remember is that like with any relationship, you may need to build trust before you can fully collaborate. As you try these statements, see if you notice what feels supportive to your inner child, and use that as a template to continue the conversation.

- I'm sorry I haven't been listening. I am listening now.
- It was not your fault.
- It's okay to make mistakes.
- You matter. You've always mattered.
- I won't leave you.
- I will set the boundaries needed for safety.
- You don't have to do it all. We can ask for help now.
- You will not be enough for everyone. But you are enough for me.
- Your _____ (fear, anger, anxiety, sadness, etc.) makes sense. I will help you feel this emotion and/or find safety.
- It's okay to feel sad (lonely, anxious, frustrated, etc.).
- Your "no" matters to me.
- I want to hear what you have to say.
- You don't have to be perfect.
- Can I show you how things are different now?
- How can I show you that I love you?
- What did you need in _____ situation that you didn't get?
- You are beloved.

7. On page 73 of *Try Softer*, I introduce a chart that helps us understand how our bodies and experiences are affected as we go into hyperarousal (fight/flight/fawn), as well as into hypoarousal (freeze/dissociation). Now I invite you to assess your experiences with hyper- and hypoarousal and fill out the chart based on your unique experiences.

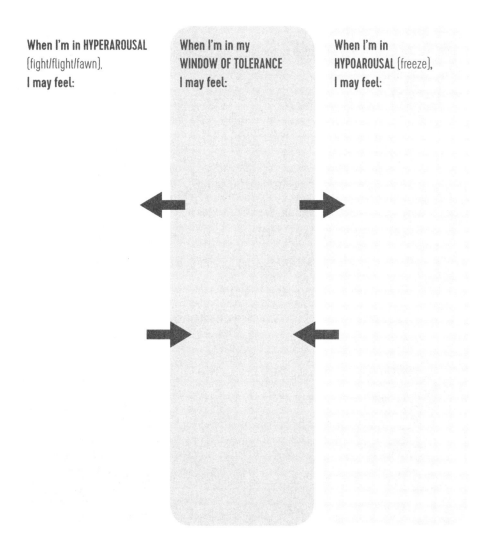

When I'm in HYPERAROUSAL
(fight/flight/fawn),
I may feel:

When I'm in my
WINDOW OF TOLERANCE
I may feel:

When I'm in
HYPOAROUSAL (freeze),
I may feel:

8. When you feel in control, grounded, curious, and content, do you believe your window of tolerance (WOT) is small or big? What are some of the experiences, relationships, or resources that contribute to its size?

9. As you consider your WOT, do you find you have a high tolerance in some situations and not in others? What differences can you observe between these situations? Take a moment to write down what you notice.

10. What practices in your life help you stay connected to your WOT?

INVITATION TO JOURNAL

How would you describe your inner child? What characteristics do you have? Are you silly? Reserved? What are your hopes and dreams?[8]

Write a letter to your inner child from the perspective of the parent you wish you'd had. Tell your inner child what you love about them. What do you hope your inner child will believe deep in their bones?

Do you believe God sees you as His beloved? Hearing that term applied in this way, what emotions does it bring up? Spend time reflecting with the Lord about why your beloved-ness matters to Him, and what would make you feel that kind of love. If you find it difficult to believe that you are God's beloved, I invite you to consider someone you love and how God thinks of them. Is it possible to allow yourself to sit alongside that person in receiving God's love for you? What do you notice as you sit alongside this person? Can you name any emotions or sensations? Finally, consider whether you have ever had a moment of time—even a glimpse—when it felt true. I invite you to write about that time. Spend a moment sitting with this as you feel able.

CONNECTION WITH GOD

& OTHERS IS THE

CURRENCY THAT ALLOWS

EACH OF US TO EXPERIENCE

COREGULATION.

INVITATION TO CREATE

On page 64 of *Try Softer*, there is a list of Scriptures for building a safe attachment with God. Read through them with your inner child in mind. Which one resonates most deeply? Which one resonates least? As you consider these, take a moment to visualize and ask your inner child what is needed in order to believe these verses are true. For now, you may simply write any response you hear in the space below. Or you may consider assuring your inner child that you are hearing what they are saying.

Next, in a grounded space, spend time creating a depiction of the Scripture with which you resonate most deeply. Whether it's rewriting it with colored pens or using watercolors to abstractly represent how it makes you feel, spend some time creating with the Lord, listening to what He has to say as you uniquely engage with His Word.

Strengthening Your Container

On pages 87–88 of *Try Softer*, I introduce what's known as a containment exercise. I invite you to take a moment and recall the container you previously created, or take a moment and create one now. As a reminder, you can be as creative as possible with your container. For example, I've had clients pick many extraordinary ideas that worked for them—everything from a fire that burns up their distress to the hands of God holding their pain to a rocket ship that takes their disturbance away. I share these examples because the most important element of the container is that it works *for you*.

With your container in mind, take some time to draw a picture of it. Feel free to add as much detail, as much color, as many quotes, and as many other elements as necessary to make it most salient for you. If it feels helpful, you may also consider creating multiple containers. Sometimes when a disturbance feels more overwhelming, we may start with one container and then put that first container into additional containers until we can notice in our body that we have the amount of "space" we need in order to take a break from the hard. Like a craftsman fashions a Russian babushka[9] doll with multiple layers, you can add additional layers to your containment exercise. Ultimately the goal is to empower you to have choices about when and how you choose to work on those elements you've had to place into the container in the first place.

BOUNDARIES ARE

THE DISTANCE AT

WHICH I CAN LOVE

YOU & ME

SIMULTANEOUSLY.

PRENTIS HEMPHILL

THE LIMITS THAT FREE US

A Deeper Dive into Chapters 5 and 6 of *Try Softer*

KAT ARRIVED IN MY OFFICE AND PLOPPED DOWN ON MY COUCH. We'd always had a fun banter that I enjoyed as her therapist. After saying hello, she began to tell me what was on her mind. We'd been working together for about six months, especially around the fawn response and boundary issues that seemed to continually cause her to experience anxiety and then later resentment.

"Here's what I don't understand," Kat explained. "With several people in my life, I've actually become really good at setting boundaries. It feels like such a relief when I say something and I know they will respect it—even if they don't like it or agree. I've noticed when I spend time around those people—the ones who honor and listen to my boundaries—it makes trying softer so much easier. It's like for the first time in my life I can actually tell what my body needs, even when I'm in the presence of others."

"But, do you remember my friend Gwen?" Kat asked.

"I do," I replied, encouraging her to continue.

Kat and I had done quite a bit of boundary work addressing a friendship that caused her significant distress. Kat had shared with me that Gwen reminded her of her mother, and Gwen often made fun of Kat or became passive-aggressive after Kat set a boundary.

"Well, I saw her last weekend—and honestly, I noticed how much harder it was to stay in touch with myself because I was worried about her the whole time. After we finished hanging out, she sent me a super-hurtful text. She told me she's 'sick of my boundaries' and doesn't know why I'm so high-maintenance."

As Kat shared this with me, pain crossed her face, and her lip quivered. This had, in fact, been an incredibly similar experience to the ones she'd had in her family growing up.

As Kat and I continued to process her concerns and validate the pain she was experiencing, I also took a moment to reframe why boundaries matter so much.

"The thing is, Kat, you're not doing anything wrong. You've been incredibly brave with Gwen. It makes sense that boundaries are hard, given your history with your family. But I'm wondering if we could reframe your 'why' behind setting your boundaries. Perhaps instead of feeling like you have to protect yourself from others, you could look at boundaries as the desire to create enough safety so you can continue to try softer.

"In a way, this boundary work we're doing now is like a love letter to your younger self, who never had those boundaries. As you lean into this work while staying attuned to the parts of you that are hurting, you're reminding those hurting parts of yourself that they matter."

The room was quiet. Kat exhaled as a few tears trickled down her cheeks.

Finally Kat looked up at me and said, "You're right, Aundi. I love Gwen, but this isn't okay. And I'm realizing what's worse is that when I feel so unsafe, there's no way for me to go deeper into my own work."

At the core of boundary work is learning to honor and respond to our need for emotional, physical, spiritual, and relational safety. And while safety and compassionate attention may not necessarily seem like they're connected, they're actually deeply intertwined. As Kat discussed above, when her body felt safe, she was better able to listen and respond to what was actually going on emotionally and spiritually within her.

I can't help but wonder if this is why in Psalm 16:6, David praises God, saying, "The boundary lines have fallen for me in pleasant places" (NIV). So many of us can relate to the settledness that comes when we know the boundary lines are where they need to be, because this is the place where we feel safe enough to turn inward or outward as we need.

As you read these words from Psalm 16, what do you notice in your body? For me, I feel the sense of a great big exhale, a sense that God is with me, and a sense that while I have the responsibility of what God has given me to do, I don't need to do more than that. I am not God (thank goodness), so I can be responsible for and faithful to what's in front of me—nothing more and nothing less.

Yet it takes tremendous courage to live within the limits our Creator sets for us, doesn't it? Honoring the reality of our finite humanity is brave work. Not only that, but for many of us, events of our childhood or other overwhelming experiences have wired our bodies to respond to life as though everything *were* our responsibility to fix. My hope for our continued work is that you will have what you need to attune to the information and responses your body provides for you as you move more deeply into boundaries and compassionate attention.

BODY-CENTERED EXERCISE

To delve more deeply into the ways boundaries and trying softer weave together, I invite you to practice a visualization that utilizes both attentional control and psychological boundaries.[1]

To begin, find a comfortable position, either seated or standing. Bring your awareness to your posture, and see if you can strengthen your core. As you do, notice the ground underneath your body. Observe where your body ends and where the space around it begins. Notice how much space you take up in the room. Observe your breath as you begin to center your body and ground yourself in the space. Then recall an issue or a person with whom you've had difficulty maintaining a boundary (as always, be mindful of your limits, and know you can discontinue this exercise if needed). See whether you can visualize this issue or person in another part of the world—separate from you. Now, simply observe what it feels like to acknowledge this issue or person, knowing you don't have to do anything else.

Next, consider a color that feels helpful, healing, or protective to you. In your mind's eye, visualize a bubble surrounding you that keeps you from being overwhelmed by this person or issue. Observe that you can make the bubble wider or smaller. Take a moment to be curious about what feels best to you. Now bring your attention back to your body, and notice what it's like to have more separateness from this person or issue. If it's helpful, recall the Scripture verse below as you sit in this space of safety:

> Lord, you alone are my portion and my cup;
>   you make my lot secure.
> The boundary lines have fallen for me in pleasant places.
> PSALM 16:5-6, NIV

Remain in this place for as long as is helpful for you, remembering you can utilize this additional boundary anytime you need to.

SIMPLE WAYS TO STATE A BOUNDARY

1. "Thanks so much for asking, but I'm not available."

2. "Sorry, that won't work for me."

3. "I'm not comfortable with that—I think I'll pass."

4. "You can handle it however works best for you, but count me out."

5. "No."

INVITATION TO REFLECT AND DISCUSS

1. Part of chapter 5 explores what the Bible—specifically Jesus—has to say about boundaries, and while Jesus suffered because of others, "He lived out this truth from a place of choice—not because He was shamed into it" (page 95 of *Try Softer*). How does this new perspective of Jesus change how you view setting limits?

2. Most of us have trouble setting limits—with ourselves, with our time, with the people around us. What are some of the reasons that keep you from setting boundaries? Where do you notice it in your body when you feel unable to hold a boundary?

3. When have you overidentified with your emotions? What was the result?

4. Think about a normal day for you. Now describe what your day would look like if you attended to yourself with compassionate attention throughout. How would you talk to yourself? What would you notice? How would you talk to others?

5. Mindfulness is a practice that can be difficult (but possible) to cultivate. Where in your life do you already feel most mindful? Where do you feel least? Is there any wisdom from the area of your life where you are already mindful you can share with the part of your life that feels the least mindful?

6. As we know, our bodies keep the score of our pains and hypervigilance. When you are overobservant of those around you (as opposed to cultivating attention to your own inner world), what does that feel like?

7. Attuning can be such a powerful force of safety in a relationship. What does it feel like when someone fully attunes to you? Is there a relationship you could cultivate more attunement in? If so, who is that relationship with?

8. What does it mean to you to love your neighbor *as yourself*? How does that change how you view yourself—and how does it change your actions?

9. Do you resonate with the description of the *fawn response* on pages 26 and 93 of *Try Softer*? Why or why not? In what ways has the fawn response affected how you set boundaries?

10. What is one boundary you may need to set in your life? What would it look like to take a step toward setting that today?

AT THE CORE OF BOUNDARY WORK

IS LEARNING TO HONOR

AND RESPOND TO

OUR NEED FOR EMOTIONAL,

PHYSICAL, SPIRITUAL

& RELATIONAL SAFETY.

INVITATION TO JOURNAL

Describe an experience where you didn't feel like you held your boundaries. Note what the situation felt like in your body, what you were thinking during the interaction, and how the person you were interacting with responded. How did you feel after the experience?

Now describe an experience where you were able to assert your needs and hold a necessary boundary. How did it feel in your body to listen to what your body and soul needed—and to ask for it? How did you feel after the experience?

INVITATION TO CREATE

Much of the rhythm of learning to try softer is about giving ourselves permission to turn with compassion to those things that are hard (e.g., boundaries), but also—and this is important—giving ourselves permission to be filled with goodness as we're able. We need both. In a sense, it is the goodness that gives us what we need to face the hard.

In this section, I invite you to deepen your well of goodness through a more robust practice of beauty hunting, as described on pages 128–30 of *Try Softer*. To begin, I invite you to explore a place or an object that feels beautiful *to you*. Remember, beauty is subjective and more full than any glossy magazine or perfect Pinterest project could capture.

As always, you can choose how to make beauty hunting work best for you. But to strengthen our practice, I invite you to take a walk or a hike or to ride somewhere you've never been before. As you do this, challenge yourself to zoom in on small details. What do you notice? Have the trees lost their leaves? What do the shapes of the bare branches look like? Do you see frost on grass? Does ice or water glisten? Can you hear ice crunch? How are the rocks shaped? What is the texture of the ground? Next, zoom out to take in the whole scene. What is the color scheme? What is unique about this place? What sensations do these things evoke in you?

Now, take either a mental picture or an actual picture of something you may want to re-create from this place. Like all our exercises, you can adapt this step to what works for you. You may want to use watercolors or colored pencils, or even cutout pictures from magazines, to evoke what you experienced.

THE WORD BECAME

FLESH AND BLOOD,

AND MOVED INTO

THE NEIGHBORHOOD.

JOHN 1:14, MSG

TENDING OUR FULL HUMANITY

A Deeper Dive into Chapters 7 and 8 of *Try Softer*

IN THE SPAN OF JUST FOUR MONTHS during a difficult season of navigating a pandemic, Brendan and I lost three members of our extended family. Two dear uncles and one beloved grandma, to be exact. It was a time of deep grief.

Though I know a lot about emotional health, what it means to care for our bodies, and the hope of heaven—these losses hit me. Hard. In part, because grief can be complicated, and it seemed to just keep coming. Additionally, everything felt harder because these waves of grief were coming in the middle of a global pandemic when everything already felt hard.

The afternoon I found out about my grandma's death, I thought to myself naively, *This will be hard, but you knew this grief was coming. It will be okay.* Somewhere in the back of my mind I also imagined that since I had already experienced much pain in this life, maybe I wouldn't feel this loss as much.

And, it was okay eventually. But first I had to grieve. I had to let the waves of emotion move through my body and process all that it meant to lose someone I love. In a real way, I had to intentionally try softer with my body and my emotions once again. This act of tenderness was the gateway toward allowing my body to begin to metabolize the pain. Frankly, this was an act of courage for me. Like so many other times before, the intense season of life I was in caused me to want to white-knuckle it or check out in so many ways. Yet my truest self knew what I most needed was compassion for the aches of my soul.

Later on that same afternoon when I found out about my grandma, the real story of my grief unfolded. After a short walk, where I listened to worship music, I noticed the achiness and weight in my chest. At that point I had not yet cried, which felt curious to me, but I wanted to simply honor my own process. Then as the late summer air rustled the trees, I envisioned my grandma breathing her last and being received into Jesus' arms. And finally, the tears began to flow.

As my body moved, my whole self processed the bigness and the fullness of this loss. And not just this one, but all the ambiguous losses that were tied up in the bizarre season the world was in.

In *Try Softer*, I include one of my favorite stories about Jesus. The way He weeps with His dear friends Mary and Martha, even though He would soon raise Lazarus, moves me. And though we can know about Jesus' show of emotion cognitively and even feel positive toward it, many of us have learned, either implicitly or explicitly, that our bodies are bad—and our emotions are too.

Yet Jesus is constantly pointing us to the truer story of our humanity. He is showing us how to move more deeply into our God-given humanness. In her important book *Walking on Water*, Madeleine L'Engle says this: "As Christians we are meant to be not less human than other people but more human, just as Jesus of Nazareth was more human."[1]

Jesus teaches us to be alive in light of the magnificent love of our Creator. Paradoxically, learning to be fully alive and human means we move toward letting ourselves feel the full range of emotions and sensations.

I share this knowing that for some of you, it's not as simple as just letting yourself feel. If it were, I don't think you'd be reading this today and journeying alongside me. You have, perhaps, faced situations that felt so overwhelming and disturbing that merely considering them now can cause your body to move into hypervigilance or a desire to be numb. You have also, perhaps, lived through situations that others have told you were "not that bad," but as you've investigated them further, you've come to realize they were disturbing *for you*. None of these experiences of pain make you weak, inferior, or lacking in faith. Instead, this information from your body simply tells you when you need to be exceptionally gentle with yourself as you experience these God-given emotions.

So this is where the compassion comes in: As we bring our curiosity and compassion to the stories of our bodies, our bodies will begin to communicate what else they need. As with so much of the work that we do to try softer, we rest in paradox. We rest in knowing that sometimes all we can know is the next step; and yet that next step is vital.

For me, in my own journey of stewarding my emotions and body, the invitation to reframe them as an ally and a gift continues to deepen. My hope and prayer for you, dear one, is that you will hold this same invitation with an open heart. You may not yet consider your body and emotions an ally, but perhaps you can begin to respect how they've worked to serve you.

BODY-CENTERED EXERCISE

In this exercise, we are going to continue to cultivate respect for the way our bodies have served us. From a grounded space, I invite you to sit or stand in a comfortable position. As you do, choose a part of your body for which you feel gratitude or respect. For example, could you thank your legs for holding you up? Your mouth for allowing you to taste? Your heart for helping you to feel and be human?

For me, I have begun to thank my belly for holding three babies, two of whom are on this earth. When I practice this exercise, I place my hands on my belly and say, "Thank you for the work you've done." As you feel able, I invite you to practice this exercise, placing your hands on any part of your body that you're extending gratitude toward.

Next, take a moment to see how that part of your body is responding toward your respect and/or gratitude. As a reminder, if this becomes overwhelming or difficult, you may consider starting with a part of your body that you feel neutral toward. For example, if you feel neutral about your feet, you could begin by thanking your feet for all the hard work they've done to carry you and bear weight. As with any practice, you'll want to be aware of your window of tolerance.

INVITATION TO REFLECT AND DISCUSS

1. Growing up, what were you taught about your body? How has that shaped what you believe about your body and other bodies now?

2. Are there any activities you have practiced now or in the past where you have felt fully present in your body?

3. Have you long believed that mind over matter is the way to get in shape and get things done? If so, what results have you seen? Where has this age-old notion been challenged?

4. After learning how Jesus values not only the spiritual but also the physical, what does an embodied faith look like to you?

5. What is one way you can practice embodiment today?

6. On page 166 of *Try Softer*, I list common statements we may have been taught about feelings. Which one, if any, resonates with your experience the most? When you sense shame toward your feelings or an urge to minimize or dismiss your emotions, do you feel that anywhere in your body (e.g., tightness in your chest, racing heart, etc.)? What are some supportive ways you can combat this trend of criticizing your emotions?

7. Have your emotions ever made an experience come alive, where they were actually a *strength* of the situation as opposed to a weakness? Summarize that experience here.

8. Using the feelings chart below, take a moment to consider where you experience different emotions in your body. As you're able, make a note on the following page about what you notice.

LIST OF FEELINGS

Nearly fifty years ago, psychologist Paul Ekman identified six emotions he said are shared by people in every culture. The list below starts with those basic emotions and then provides many more gradations.

Happy	Sad	Angry	Fearful	Surprised	Disgusted
Amused	Blue	Aggravated	Afraid	Astonished	Cynical
Carefree	Burdened	Agitated	Alarmed	Confused	Disillusioned
Cheerful	Depressed	Bitter	Antsy	Curious	Disturbed
Excited	Despondent	Brooding	Anxious	Delighted	Embarrassed
Exhilarated	Disappointed	Cranky	Brooding	Enchanted	Exasperated
Giddy	Discouraged	Cross	Cautious	Horrified	Fed Up
Grateful	Drained	Defensive	Despairing	Impressed	Humiliated
Joyful	Gloomy	Frustrated	Frightened	Incredulous	Jaded
Loved	Grief-stricken	Furious	Helpless	Inquisitive	Jealous
Merry	Hopeless	Hostile	Hesitant	Intrigued	Offended
Optimistic	Lonely	Impatient	Insecure	Mystified	Outraged
Relaxed	Melancholic	Rebellious	Nervous	Puzzled	Repulsed
Satisfied	Pensive	Resentful	Rattled	Shocked	Revolted
Thrilled	Remorseful	Scorned	Stressed	Skeptical	Scandalized
Tranquil	Troubled	Testy	Tense	Startled	Sickened
Upbeat	Weary	Upset	Worried	Wary	Smug

9. What does it feel like for you to be in emotional overwhelm? What about disconnection? Write about a circumstance that created the need for you to go into overwhelm or disconnection. What would it be like to approach that experience from a more grounded space?

INVITATION TO JOURNAL

As an extension of the body-centered exercise earlier in this session, write a letter to your body. See if you can view your body through a lens of compassionate attention. Consider the ways that your body has carried you, helped you to function, and allowed you to survive. Take a moment to honor and acknowledge the pain, harm, or intensity that has been sustained by your body.

When do you love your body the most? When has your body felt most like itself?

Write the story of your body—your first memories of your body, the trials and tribulations you've been through together, how you feel about it now. What does your body need to hear from you today?

Like David, we, too, can pour our hearts out to God. Write out a psalm expressing what emotions you have during this season of your life.

On page 170 of *Try Softer*, I describe how emotions and feelings are similar, yet different: Emotions speak to the sensations in the body—but feelings are what we name those sensations. Take a moment to acknowledge how your emotions begin to shift into feelings. (For example, when I read a tender story, I may notice a sensation of tingling and fullness around my eyes. Initially I may recognize that I'm feeling a sense of sadness. But as I become more curious about my emotions, I have a chance to unpack that the particular story I'm reading brings up feelings of nostalgia, grief, and bittersweet hope.) See if you can see the evolution from emotional sensations to feelings in your own body. As you're able, take a moment to write about what you notice.

JESUS IS CONSTANTLY

POINTING US

TO THE TRUER STORY

OF OUR HUMANITY.

INVITATION TO CREATE

So often what we think about ourselves is different from how others perceive us. In this section, I invite you to create a self-portrait that reflects how someone who cares about you may view you. If you're able and you so choose, you could make yourself the person who cares about you. If that feels too challenging, consider who else would see you with a kind gaze. This could be your child, God, a spouse, a friend, a therapist, a pastor, or any other supportive person.

As a reminder, there's no need to be an artist here. The more important element of this exercise is giving yourself permission to tap into your right-brain creativity and processing.

A few other questions to keep in mind as you are creating include the following:

· How can you reflect your strengths in the portrait? Your battle scars? Your fire? (Those things that bring out your passion and advocacy.)

· What do you notice about how you feel as you're creating this portrait?

· What part of your portrait do you feel most connected to?

TALK TO
YOURSELF LIKE YOU
WOULD TO SOMEONE
YOU LOVE.

BRENÉ BROWN

INHABITING OUR BELOVEDNESS

A Deeper Dive into Chapters 9 and 10 of Try Softer

PERHAPS ONE OF THE MOST COMMON AREAS of pushback I hear about trying softer is the fear that if we begin to cultivate compassionate attention for ourselves—especially with parts like our inner critics—we'll become lazy, selfish, or incompetent.

> "What if I'm kind to myself and I don't change?" one reader wondered.

> "How about if I'm too compassionate and I stay stuck?" another client feared.

> "What if I prove my parents right and show that I am worthless?" another young woman wrestled.

These questions are so common, and I often think of them when I write or speak because I know they are just on the surface, waiting to rise. Frankly, I completely understand this reticence most of us feel when we consider compassionate attention.

It's as though we fear that compassion will get out of control and we won't become who God created us to be. The paradox of compassion is that though we believe it will keep us stuck, it actually opens the door to resilience. When we recognize the astounding power of God's loving-kindness, we can finally connect to the resources that allow us to move through hardship rather than be defined by it. One of my favorite invitations for this work comes from Jesus in Matthew 11:28-30. He says it this way in *The Message* paraphrase:

Are you tired? Worn out? Burned out on religion? Come to me. Get away with me and you'll recover your life. I'll show you how to take a real rest. Walk with me and work with me—watch how I do it. Learn the unforced rhythms of grace. I won't lay anything heavy or ill-fitting on you. Keep company with me and you'll learn to live freely and lightly.

I can just imagine the folks of Jesus' day worrying about the troubles and hardship of their time and—in the midst of those difficulties—hearing Jesus' invitation. I wonder whether they asked the same questions we do: *Will there be enough? Does God care? Do I matter? Am I seen?*

And here is Jesus' utterly simple answer to the complexity of many of our questions: "Come to me. Get away with me. . . . Learn the unforced rhythms of grace."

You see, God as revealed in Jesus is the author of compassionate attention and gentleness. God, in the most infinite wisdom that could exist, knows our psyche, neurobiology, and physiology. And because this is true,

God invites us to the next step in our journey toward wholeness: connection. We are beckoned to connect with ourselves, with others, and with our Creator. God invites us to lay down our exhaustion and weariness—not to shame us, but to *meet* us.

———

Perhaps as you read this, you're nodding along, because you, too, believe God longs to meet us in our fragile, resilient, and beloved humanity. But what does it mean to truly practice it? *How?* is always the question so many of us come back to asking. The best I can tell you is to keep your eyes open for the upside-down Kingdom of Jesus. Keep your eyes open for the ways you are being invited to go deeper into your own journey.

For example, I have found that working with my own inner critic is often paradoxical. I used to think I should just tell my critic to "knock it off." And certainly I don't advocate for speaking to ourselves badly. But I've come to learn that my own personal internal critic becomes activated when I feel vulnerable. This part of myself appears when I perceive I'm experiencing some sort of danger. As a kiddo, I learned that if I am harder on myself than anyone else, people won't have to criticize me. I would think, *I can take care of that myself.*

But the upside-down economy of Jesus has taught me something different: to embrace and honor the story my body holds. So now when I notice my own personal critic getting activated, I have learned to respond like this: *Thank you for trying to protect me, but I am an adult now with different resources. I don't need to shame or berate myself anymore to belong.*

Dear reader, your inner critic or your sense of shame around not "being enough" may look different from mine. Yet my hope is you will embrace the dance of honoring your past while staying open to the new story God invites you to participate in. May you come to find that the heartbeat of God is with you and in you as you embrace this journey.

77

BODY-CENTERED EXERCISE

To engage a body-centered exercise, you may wish to consider a time when you have successfully practiced self-compassion, as described on pages 196–99 of *Try Softer*. As you recall these circumstances, how you handled them, and how it felt to give yourself permission to be imperfect and flawed, observe what you notice in your body. You may also wish to consider whether it would be helpful to bring someone into your visualization who might encourage you as you practice self-compassion. This could be a real person or a character from a book, movie, play, etc.

Alternately, if you don't recall a time you were able to practice self-compassion, you might try to remember a time when you were able to extend compassion to someone else in your life. Again, consider the circumstances and how the experience felt in your body. As you do this, utilize curiosity—is it possible to shift the compassion you experienced for the other person to yourself?

With either of these scenarios, notice if there is any affirming belief that comes up for you. For example, "I am in process" or "I am doing the best I can" or "One step at a time" or "Everyone makes mistakes, and that's okay." (For more ideas, see the list of affirmations on the next page.)

Now I invite you to place one hand on your heart and one on your belly in a way that feels supportive to you. If it's helpful, invite Jesus into this space with you. Notice if He says anything to you, or if it feels best to simply be with Him.

TRY SOFTER AFFIRMATIONS

- I have choices.
- I can set boundaries.
- It's okay to disappoint people.
- I am capable.
- I am loved no matter what.
- I am valuable.
- I can ask for support.
- It's okay to need help.
- My emotions give me information.
- My body supports me.
- My body gives me information.
- I am responsible for only myself.
- It's okay to take care of myself.
- This emotion is temporary.
- I am beloved.

INVITATION TO REFLECT AND DISCUSS

1. What makes paying compassionate attention to yourself most difficult for you? What resources or support might you need to practice this type of mindfulness?

2. Why is it so difficult to extend kindness to ourselves?

3. The idea that sometimes it is in surrender that we make the most progress toward healing can be a difficult one to accept. As I discuss on pages 212–13 of *Try Softer*, this can especially be true if we learned to cope with trauma through overfunctioning or if surrender has in some way been weaponized against us. While acknowledging this tension, consider whether there has ever been an experience in your life when surrender ultimately proved helpful. If not, is there a situation you're in right now where you could imagine the healing that surrendering could bring? As you're able, describe what this might look like for you.

4. How is the "try softer" definition of surrender different from our worldly definition? How does it change the way you think about releasing control of your circumstances?

Worldly Surrender   **Try Softer Surrender**

5. When do you feel most empowered and strong?

Wrap-Up Questions

1. What has been the most challenging part of delving more deeply into *Try Softer*?

2. What has been the best or most life-giving part?

3. What has been your biggest takeaway?

4. How do you see yourself integrating this work into your daily life?

INVITATION TO JOURNAL

Trista, a former client of mine, was exceptionally conscientious and kind. She was the type of person who regularly showed up early to her job and often stayed late. Trista initially began seeing me because she couldn't figure out why she experienced so much shame about articulating her needs—and how it led her to feel deeply lonely and even resentful in her relationships. However, as we began to get curious about Trista's inner dialogue, more became clear.

In one important session, Trista shared that her inner critic would often say, *No one wants to hear your voice. You talk way too much. Stop being needy.* After reflecting and processing, Trista came to realize that her critic's voice reminded her of her mother's—she was constantly demeaning Trista if she articulated any needs.

It took time, but eventually Trista was able to understand the role her inner critic played in her world: The critical voice was actually attempting to *protect* Trista from further rejection. If she didn't use her voice and express her opinions, she would have a better chance of "belonging" to her family.

This was a turning point in Trista's journey toward befriending her internal voice—with new understanding, she was able to move forward. Trista addressed her critic with compassion: *Thank you, critic, for trying to protect me. I needed it. But I'm an adult now; I'm not in my mother's care anymore. I know you're trying to help, but I won't let you abuse me with these words anymore.*

To the extent that you feel able, describe an instance or circumstance when your own inner critic was/is loud. Write about what you observe about yourself and/or the situation and what your inner critic was/is saying.

With a compassionate perspective in mind, see whether you can utilize curiosity to ask your inner critic what is underneath its critique. How does your critic respond when you ask about what it is *actually* afraid of when it criticizes you?

With the information you receive from your critic, take a moment to write out a response to that part of yourself. You may wish to remind your inner critic of several truths you now know, such as

you are an adult now;

you are fully and deeply loved by God; and

you now have new resources to help you grow.

Who does your inner critic remind you of?

Can you identify a paradoxical way your inner critic has kept you safe or allowed you to survive or succeed?

If God were to talk back to your inner critic, what do you think He would say?

As you look back on your life, can you identify where you've been resilient? As you're able, use the space below to validate or encourage your body for all the ways it has supported you and allowed you to be resilient.

How has your view of your own resilience shifted as you've worked through *Try Softer*?

What self-care practices help you tap into your resilience?

SPIRITUAL SELF-CARE

EMOTIONAL SELF-CARE

RELATIONAL SELF-CARE

PHYSICAL SELF-CARE

THE TRY SOFTER GUIDED JOURNEY

As we move toward completing our journey together, I invite you to take a moment to jot down any final thoughts on what it's been like for you to go through this guide.

THE PARADOX OF COMPASSION

IS THAT THOUGH WE BELIEVE

IT WILL KEEP US STUCK,

IT ACTUALLY OPENS THE DOOR

TO RESILIENCE.

INVITATION TO CREATE

One of the tensions of trying softer is that we are constantly grieving and celebrating. Why do we do this? Because this is the rhythm of life; this is what God often models for us—and not surprisingly, it's what allows our bodies to have what they need to heal and grow.

And so, for this final invitation to create, I invite you to gather ten to fifteen stones. Next, gather paint or markers. On as many of the stones as needed, write down those parts of your story that have been difficult, painful, or traumatic. As always, you're free to write only as much as feels helpful to you. On the additional stones, I invite you to write anything you've learned that has been helpful, healing, or supportive. You may consider ways you've experienced God differently, ways you are seeing yourself grow, ways you've been resilient, or affirmations that feel grounding to you. You may also consider painting and decorating these rocks in a way that reflects what you're writing. As always, you are free to make this work for you.

Finally, either individually or in a group, take a moment to gather and honor these stones that carry and name the hurt you've experienced. This can be done by simply acknowledging the reality that these stones exist (or have existed) and that those experiences matter. Next, move on to the stones that represent what has been helpful, healing, or supportive in your journey. As you name these resources, notice what it feels like to hold them in your hand. Observe the weight and any strength you feel having them with you.

BENEDICTION

A FEW YEARS AGO, when I finally completed my manuscript for *Try Softer*, I sat at my kitchen counter and wept with gratitude and hope. Since then, I have been humbled and amazed to watch other folks connect with their God-given hunger to be more compassionate with themselves and others.

But today as I write, I'm watching a blanket of white descend as I greet one of Colorado's first snows. My heart feels such a deep peace as I think of you, dear reader. Here is my prayer as you move forward in this courageous work:

> May you know in the depths of your soul that you are invited to participate with the triune God in the work of compassionate attention.
>
> May you come to inhabit your life, your body, your relationships, and your communities in ways you have never before dreamed.

May you who have sown in tears "reap in joy" (Psalm 126:5, KJV).

May everything that was stolen by trauma, the systems of the world, and the enemy be restored to your body, mind, and spirit.

And may each of us have eyes to see that God—the great coregulator of our bodies, minds, and souls—has always been with us, and for us.

May it be so.

With deep hope,
Aundi Kolber
OCTOBER 2020

GUIDANCE FOR GROUP LEADERS

LEARNING AND GROWING IN COMMUNITY is an essential part of what it means to be human. Yet as the old adage goes, we are both "harmed in relationship and healed in relationship." Because this is true, my hope is that folks who participate in a discussion group feel empowered to have both "a voice and a choice" in the work of trying softer, as well as self-attunement. Practicing and encouraging this compassionate posture also supports us as we seek to love our neighbors as ourselves. With this in mind, I've laid out a few recommendations for basic guidelines on how to facilitate a discussion group that seeks to integrate trauma-informed principles. As always, the group itself and the individuals within it can choose what works best. Seek to honor choice, autonomy, and self-attunement in the group by

- encouraging group members to answer or not answer questions depending on what feels helpful to them;

- encouraging group members to be aware of their own windows of tolerance and utilize skills to ground themselves if they become overwhelmed;

- encouraging group members to take breaks as needed throughout the group time in order to attune to themselves (e.g., to use the restroom, get a drink of water, have a snack);

- encouraging group members to honor each other's limits when someone chooses to not participate in part of a discussion;

- encouraging group members to seek professional care if or when the content or process of the group surpasses what the group can offer in terms of support; and

- encouraging group members to seek professional trauma-informed care if or when they find they'd like to continue to process themes that have come up in the group.

NOTES

INTRODUCTION

1. Daniel J. Siegel, *Mindsight: The New Science of Personal Transformation* (New York: Bantam Books, 2010), 107–8.

SESSION 1: THE STORIES WE HOLD IN OUR BODIES

1. All stories in this curriculum are a compilation of experiences based on various clients I have worked with throughout the years. All names and identifying details have been changed.

2. This is a fairly common idea within therapeutic settings. For another example of this type of supportive practice, see Arielle Schwartz and Barb Maiberger, *EMDR Therapy and Somatic Psychology: Interventions to Enhance Embodiment in Trauma Treatment* (New York: W. W. Norton, 2018), 91.

3. The fawn response, as first coined by therapist Pete Walker, is still a fairly new concept within the trauma field. Because this is true, more research is needed surrounding how it affects our nervous systems. Based on the hypervigilance often associated with the fawn response, I have placed fawn as being connected to the sympathetic nervous system. However, there is evidence that the fawn response may additionally include a hypoarousal response. For the purpose of this book and to be concise, I've kept it connected to the hyperarousal response.

SESSION 2: CONNECTION IS THE CURRENCY OF REGULATION

1. I more fully unpack the nuances of the window of tolerance in *Try Softer* on pages 71–79. My thoughts can be credited to work from Stephen W. Porges and Deb Dana, eds., *Clinical Applications of the Polyvagal Theory: The Emergence of Polyvagal-Informed Therapies* (New York: W. W. Norton, 2018); Dana, *The Polyvagal Theory in Therapy: Engaging the Rhythm of Regulation* (New York: W. W. Norton, 2018); Daniel J. Siegel, *Pocket Guide to Interpersonal Neurobiology: An Integrative Handbook of the Mind* (New York: W. W. Norton, 2012), 3-1–3-4; Pete Walker, *Complex PTSD: From Surviving to Thriving* (n.p.: Azure Coyote, 2014), 13.

2. Dr. Daniel Siegel notes that one of his patients called this "feeling felt" by another person. For more, see *Mindsight: The New Science of Personal Transformation* (New York: Bantam Books, 2010), 10.

3. See Siegel, *Pocket Guide to Interpersonal Neurobiology*, 20-2, 20-3.
4. See John Bowlby, *A Secure Base: Parent-Child Attachment and Healthy Human Development* (New York: Basic Books, 1988), 3–4.
5. See Siegel, *Pocket Guide to Interpersonal Neurobiology*, 20-2, 20-3.
6. See Allan N. Schore, "The Effects of Secure Attachment Relationship on Right Brain Development, Affect Regulation, and Infant Mental Health," *Infant Mental Health Journal* 22 (2001): 7–66; Allan N. Schore, "The Effects of Early Relationship Trauma on Right Brain Development, Affect Regulation, and Infant Mental Health," *Infant Mental Health Journal* 22 (2001): 201–69.
7. See Arielle Schwartz and Barb Maiberger, *EMDR Therapy and Somatic Psychology: Interventions to Enhance Embodiment in Trauma Treatment* (New York: W. W. Norton, 2018), 146–47.
8. Some readers may find they have more than one "inner child," which is totally normal. I'll be using the term *inner child* moving forward to be concise, however. Feel free to adapt this activity to make it work for you.
9. The formal name for these is *Matryoshka dolls*.

SESSION 3: THE LIMITS THAT FREE US

1. This is a fairly common meditation practice used to support folks in creating psychological and energetic boundaries. For more on the background of this practice, see Suzanne B. Friedman, *Heal Yourself with Qigong: Gentle Practices to Increase Energy, Restore Health, and Relax the Mind* (Oakland, CA: New Harbinger, 2009).

SESSION 4: TENDING OUR FULL HUMANITY

1. Madeleine L'Engle, *Walking on Water: Reflections on Faith and Art* (New York: Convergent Books, 2016), 51.

ABOUT THE AUTHOR

AUNDI KOLBER is a licensed professional counselor (LPC), writer, and speaker living in Castle Rock, Colorado. She graduated from Denver Seminary in 2008 with an MA in community counseling. Aundi is the owner of Kolber Counseling, LLC, established in 2009. She has received additional training in her specialization of trauma- and body-centered therapies, including the highly researched and regarded eye movement desensitization and reprocessing (EMDR) therapy.

Aundi is passionate about the integration of faith and psychology, as well as its significance for the church today. She has written for *Relevant*, CT Women, (in)courage, *HuffPost*, Propel Sophia, *Verily* magazine, and more. Aundi regularly speaks at local and national events, and she appears on podcasts such as *That Sounds Fun* with Annie Downs, *CXMH*, *The Upside Down Podcast*, *This Good Word with Steve Wiens*, and *Restoring the Soul*.

As a survivor of trauma and a lifelong learner, Aundi brings hard-won knowledge around the work of change, the power of redemption, and the beauty of experiencing God with us in our pain. She is happily married to her best friend, Brendan, and is the proud mom of Matia and Jude.

SPACE FOR TRYING SOFTER

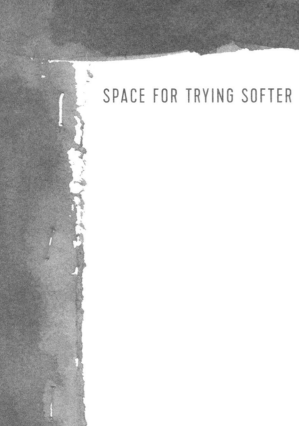

SPACE FOR TRYING SOFTER

SPACE FOR TRYING SOFTER

SPACE FOR TRYING SOFTER

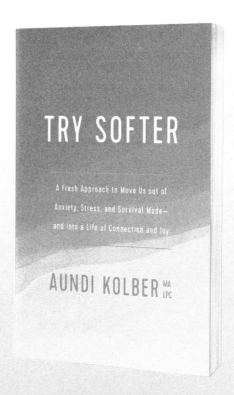